TRANSITION 2 PRACTICE

TRANSITION 2 PRACTICE

21 Things Every Doctor Must Know in Contract Negotiations and the Job Search

NAPOLEON BONAPARTE HIGGINS, JR., MD

Two Harbors Press, Minneapolis

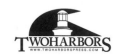

Two Harbors Press
322 First Avenue N, 5th floor
Minneapolis, MN 55401
612.455.2293
www.TwoHarborsPress.com

www.napoleonhigginsmd.com

ISBN-13: 978-1-63413-716-4
LCCN: 2015912522

Distributed by Itasca Books

Cover Design by Alan Pranke
Typeset by Colleen Rollins

Printed in the United States of America

Dedication In Memorium

To Eloise "Babe" Smith Higgins, my mother
(1943–2014)

My mother has been with me every step of the way in my life, career, and practice. As my office manager, she also served as task master for the entire office. Her mantra as mother and office manager to me as son and owner of the practice was, "Sometimes I'll let you be the boss."

My mother left me with several instructions before her passing. One was to complete this book that took longer than expected. If she were here, she would say, "As always . . . you're late!"

Mom,
Thanks for always believing in me.

About the Author

Napoleon Higgins is a child, adolescent, and adult psychiatrist who has a private practice in the Houston area. His private practice started with one physician, being himself, and his mother as his office manager. In the short period of nine years, it has become one of the largest group practices in the fourth largest city in the United States. His company, Bay Pointe Behavioral Health Service, Inc., now employs multiple clinicians, including psychiatrists, physician extenders, therapists, and supporting staff. He believes that the lack of business acumen is greatly affecting the practice and delivery of health care around the country. It is his hope that this book will help to alleviate the gap between clinical knowledge and business knowledge that is greatly lacking in the medical field. It is his belief that clinical knowledge is a major part, but not the only part, of medical education.

Contact information:
1560 W. Bay Area Blvd #110
Friendswood, TX 77546
(281) 480-240 0
www.napoleonhigginsmd.com

Acknowledgments

I would like to thank all those who have helped me along while writing this book. Many people deserve to be mentioned, but time does not allow for me to thank them all. I would be remiss if I did not thank Marilyn King and the Minority Fellowship of the American Psychiatric Association for giving me a forum to develop this topic. I also have to thank all my colleagues who have discussed their contracts and job opportunities with me. Thanks to all the doctors and staff who have worked with me at Bay Pointe Behavioral Health Service, Inc. I definitely have to acknowledge my family. God blessed me with a great family, and I had nothing to do with the selection of the people whom he placed in my life, including my mother, father, sisters, and cousins. I have to thank individually my mother, who passed before concluding this book and who supported her son through it all, and my wife, who continually puts up with all these ideas that run through my head. Oddly enough, I see that one of them actually came to fruition. A special thanks to all those who should have been mentioned but I did not name either due to forgetfulness, keeping them anonymous, or lack of couth. As the saying goes, "Charge it to my head and not my heart."

Foreword

I have met many physicians at many different phases of their careers. Most state they wish they knew more about contracts. Most will also state that their formal education of business is poor and training on how to negotiate a contract or how to find the right job is essentially nonexistent. We fail to realize that even though how much you will make financially is very important, it is just another part of negotiating the right job for you.

I've found that much legal text can be very dry and difficult to read due to legal jargon, and many physicians may get lost quickly in verbiage and boredom. This book is written so that it may be a quick and easy read for physicians who are signing an employment contract and/or looking for a job opportunity. The intent of this book is not to be a comprehensive text of negotiating contracts or finding work. This book is written with the context of what doctors most often miss in contract negotiations and finding the right job for them.

Disclaimer

This is not meant to be a legal textbook. This book does not substitute the need for a legal assistance in negotiating a contract or looking for employment. Realize that the author is a psychiatrist by trade and not a lawyer and has no formal legal training or certification in contract negotiations.

Contents

I

Physician, Know Thyself

1. Before You Negotiate: Introspection

"How can you negotiate for what you want if you don't know what you are looking for?"

What is it that you want from medicine? Why did you go into it?

These are questions you should ask yourself before deciding what type of job you want to take. How can you negotiate for what you want if you don't know what you are looking for? Before negotiating, ask the questions: Where are you now? Where do you want to be in a year, five years, twenty years, retirement? Of course, ideas may change over time, but you need to head in a direction that fits your goals. The better able you are to define what you want, the better chance you have of negotiating for the right job for you.

 Mistake: Taking a job according to what is popular with your mentors or peers.

It is similar to driving a car. If you have no particular place to go, then you drive your career aimlessly. You will eventually get lost, run out of gas, or you become an accident waiting to happen. Many of us find ourselves without direction. Some are thinking that the solution to their working problem is making more money. Many don't realize that as the Beatles said, "Money can't buy me love," nor will it buy a good career. What is more important is contentment and being able to do medicine in an environment that makes you feel productive, have direction, and be well compensated for your work. When thinking of the perfect contract and essential work environment, you should think of which job will allow you to do the work that you want to do, be respected, and have direction for your career. If you don't know what you want, it is difficult to negotiate because neither the employer nor you know what is best for you.

You should start with figuring out what your dream practice or job is. Make sure that this is practical, though. I know you want to make a million dollars a year while working twenty-four hours a week, be seen as the world expert in your field, have all the respect of your colleagues, be celebrated, appreciated, and well loved, but back to reality. What is it that is a must in your career and practice of medicine? Is it present with you where you are? You must ask yourself and answer the question: How do I get there? This is the premise of the negotiation. It starts with: What is in it for my situation and where do I want to be?

Money, Power, and Respect

In 1998 the rap group the Lox released the song "Money, Power & Respect" featuring Lil' Kim and DMX. So often in our instant-gratification twenty-first-century lifestyle, we lose the fact that hard work goes into building careers and receiving "money, power, and respect."

Example

> I once had a colleague who stated that she interviewed a child and adolescent psychiatrist who was just finishing residency and inquired about a job in her office. The resident, who had not worked independently in their job, asked for a salary at $235,000 when the average salary was $165,000 for the area. The asking salary was given with the ultimatum that the salary was not further negotiable.

Essentially, other than finishing school, the recent graduate had no other qualification to show why he deserved to be paid more than the average-peered colleagues. The issue with my friend was: Why pay someone who has not proven their worth over their value? The other question was: Why pay someone that amount when there are others who have proven themselves and are available for the same amount or less? There is no need to say that the offer for employment was withdrawn.

Many people do not realize what it takes to establish a well-renowned or highly paid career. Building a career obviously takes time, but also you have to remember that all buildings are done by design. It really takes hard work and dedication to a field or area to develop yourself. Being a physician is hard enough, but you have to go beyond the normal busy and hectic call of duty for a physician. It is rare for luck to strike an individual's career, but even if it does, it is required to strike again and again in order to maintain. If you ask most people who are deemed "successful" by physicians how they got to their position, most will tell you that hard work and an opportunity occurred where they could put their abilities on display. This is not only true in medicine but in all professions. Remember, though, if you do not put in the hard work, you will not able to seize the opportunity when present. If you do seize an opportunity without hard work, then it will be difficult to sustain the success.

You Doc, Inc.

"You take your knowledge and skills with you wherever you go."

Remember that your greatest asset and benefit to any company is what is in your head. This comes through your training. You take your knowledge and skills with you wherever you go. It doesn't matter the time, place, or situation. You have to understand that the information you know is world class and difficult to attain. The skills are critically needed. It would take a genius at least ten years to have what you possess by the time you finish your training. In fact, most medical doctors are going to have very high IQs and many are geniuses.

Due to our skills traveling with us, we have the opportunity to find employment just about anywhere because everywhere there is a need for a doctor. Every doctor receives job opportunities constantly with people attempting to lure them away from where they are working. So, if you are unhappy where you are working and have other options, then why are you still working there?

Your work should be about you. Corporate bodies think of themselves and see you as a commodity. It is great to be on a job where they appreciate you and deem you a very necessary part of the treatment team. As physicians, we are dedicated to our patients, staff, and treatment team. We find ourselves working in units and gaining camaraderie over time. All this may be true, but what happens if the bottom line isn't met by a medical entity? What occurs when they find the need to save on salaries and cut services that are not as productive? If they need to cut a physician and the dollars and cents say that cutting you will make things more profitable, then you should expect to be cut.

 Conclusion: You must understand who you are and what you want before beginning to negotiate in your best interest. Introspection is key to the negotiation. The ultimate dream job can become a nightmare if you take a job in what is someone else's best interest and not your own.

2. All Things Are Negotiable

It is important to understand that you are always negotiating. Many of these are conscious decisions, such as determining how much we are willing to pay for a house or whether it is worth an additional twenty cents for caramel syrup on a double chocolate macchiato. You negotiate everything from when to wake up in the morning to the route you are going to take to work. You negotiate where you will stop for gas based upon what side of the street you are on when you go to work and what you are going to eat for lunch that day based on menu options. Many of these decisions are based on convenience, price, or familiarity. Like such, we negotiate whether to take a job both consciously and unconsciously.

 Mistake: Taking a great job and believing that the details will work themselves out.

Many times when a physician negotiates a contract, they have no idea what the process entails. We often may believe that the type of contract we are negotiating is non-negotiable. We will think that because this is a large entity (e.g., hospital, government agency, or university), we cannot negotiate with them. The problem this represents is that a physician may pass on a good opportunity because there are things in the contract that they do not like or certain terms they do not feel comfortable with. This poses an issue with the employer in that a person may not join the organization over something that could have been worked out if there was adequate negotiating.

Location

We have all seen the job inquiry that states:

LOCATED WITHIN AN HOUR OF A MAJOR
COLLEGE UNIVERSITY

FOUR SEASONS

EXCELLENT FISHING

EXCELLENT SCHOOLS

NEAR FOUR LAKES

WITHIN TWO HOURS OF A MAJOR
PRESIDENTIAL LIBRARY

LOW COST OF LIVING

STARTING SALARY OF A GAZILLION DOLLARS

Typically, if you see something like this and the town, city, or state is not mentioned, then you assume you are going to be in the middle of nowhere. This is an example just to show you how we often make our decisions on negotiating unconsciously. If you desire to be in a small town that is an hour away from a small city, then this may be a place for you. Or if you are used to living in a major metropolis, you may decide it is not for you. Some people may feel this is a great opportunity to make money for a few years and pay off medical school loans. Others may feel this may be an escape from the metropolitan lifestyle and think this will be an excellent place to get away, raise kids, and settle down at a slower pace. Some may even find it is an excellent place to practice medicine as part of the witness protection program.

Make sure to consider workload, responsibilities, ancillary staff, benefits packages, and overall compensation for the job. It is possible to be in a rural small town, at a small hospital, with a very small ancillary staff and at the same time be a medical hub for a very large catchment area in a rural place. This can be busier than working in a large urban hospital in a university setting placed in the middle of a metropolis. Some of the best doctors I have met are away from the public and academic eye, working and grinding it out every day without any recognition outside of their local community that they have been working in for decades. We as doctors often make these assumptions based on a very limited amount of information given by a recruitment firm or on first glance of a small flyer or ad in our professional journals. This goes to say that we make quick judgments and negotiate jobs all the time.

Salary

"It is difficult to go up on a requested salary once you have given a salary amount."

Most salaries are not set in stone. When negotiating salary, it is natural that the most common thought is to negotiate for more. Realize that you may have been offered a very handsome salary and a potential employer might be perturbed that you would ask for more. It can come off as unappreciative and arrogant, especially if you do not have factual numbers to suggest why you deserve the amount you are asking for. Of course it is also possible to undershoot and cheat yourself. It is difficult to go up on a requested salary once you have given a salary amount.

Remember that salary should be comparable to the service that is to be done. Make sure you inquire about salaries for other doctors in the area who do similar work. Your salary should be comparative to people with similar education, credentials, board certifications, years of experience, and level of expertise.

You typically should not be surprised by the salary amount. Based on the description of the job and researching the salary information before you interview, you should be pretty close to knowing the amount before the actual number is given. If you feel the salary offered is too low, remember it is best to negotiate with factual numbers when asking for a higher salary. These numbers should be based on the research you have done.

There are multiple sites on the Internet that will give you the information you need on salaries. Some of those include:

- www.salary.com
- www.payscale.com
- www.glassdoor.com
- www.bls.gov
- www.salaryexpert.com

Also remember that many public hospitals publish this information, and a ten-minute search online will give you the exact base salary that others make at a particular institution.

If the employer overpays for the service, then you run the risk of being laid off, or rather the first cut in downsizing. If the salary you desire is less than you expected, it is essential to mention this and ask for an explanation. You want to make sure you are "comparing apples to apples."

It is possible to negotiate more profitable work into your schedule in order to justify the higher salary. Potential employers want to know if it is profitable for you to be on staff. If you can show this in hard numbers, then it is more likely that you will be able to make the case for the higher salary. This works if it is mutually beneficial to both the potential employer and employee.

 Conclusion: It is important to understand that you are always negotiating, whether consciously or unconsciously. It is important to make as many conscious decisions as possible in picking the right job and contract for you.

3. Negotiate to Win

"You are trying to find a job that fits you as an employee, and the employer is trying to find the right employee for the job."

We often think of negotiations as if it is based on either "I win" or "you lose." The ideal, though, is that we both win, as discussed in the book by Jim Thomas, *Negotiate to Win*. Yes, that is correct; the best negotiations are based on both parties winning. We also often think of negotiations as we see them on television dramas or the news about high-stakes talks between Israel and Palestine or the United States negotiating with the Taliban. When going into negotiating regarding a job, let's "take it down a thousand." Realize what it is for what it is. You are trying to find a job that fits you as an employee, and the employer is trying to find the right employee for the job.

 Mistake: Believing that a company is too big and that you are too small to negotiate.

I Lose; They Win

This is never an ideal situation for most people who are going to read this book. If you take a job where you feel you are losing, you will find yourself disgruntled on the job, which can really hurt your morale on the job and hurt the morale of the people having to work with you. The question is: Why are you losing? Did you know that you were going to be at a loss before taking the job? If so, why are you considering the job? At this point, it is important to do some introspection, either with why are you considering a job you don't want or why are you in a job you don't like? There are times when you simply made a mistake and did not consider all the factors, or you could know the job is temporary and is the means to an end. You will find the less-than-ideal job as a necessity and tolerable if you know there is an end point to the suffering.

I Win; They Lose

Losing for the other party can also still be stressful on the employee who felt like they won. This could make for a bad work environment for the winner. Often what you find is that this can bring contention in the workplace. If an employer believes they are overcompensating for the work provided, then the employer may be looking at the employee as an unnecessary expenditure. This means the employee could be the first to be let go in case of downsizing. I often hear of people coming on a job and making more money and having more benefits than those who have the same credentials, proven productivity, and longer tenure on the job. If those people find out someone of lesser value is making more than they are, this can be very disruptive and cause a disgruntled workplace. Also, people may be unwilling to work collegially with the new overpaid employee.

I Lose; They Lose

This leaves both parties miserable and is the ultimate setup for a situation that is not going to work out. The question is: How did both the employer and employee get into a mutually bad situation? Either one or the other misrepresented themselves, there was a lack of communication regarding the job, or the job was poorly defined on what it entailed. These relationships are the worst and require careful evaluation on how it got to that point. Most likely the employment will not last much longer if an agreement cannot be worked out. Both parties may be in a situation where they are both thinking it is an ends to a mean. After consideration of how both got there, see if there is something redeemable about the situation and attempt to work it out in a positive way where both can benefit. If not, start looking for an out.

I Win; They Win

Ideally, both parties will win. When this occurs, everyone is happy. Also know that this is possible and happens more often than some would expect. You want to be at a job where you are appreciated and respected for what you bring to a company. You will find that you will work harder on a job that you like and that develops your career.

Realize that any situation that is not a win-win is a lose-lose. This is not television where hostile takeovers are the norm and one party walks off with billions while the others are left penniless. This happens, but it's not very often. Also, you must realize that what a doctor is looking for and an employer desires is typically not high-stakes television drama. At least it is not for most of us. The point is to come to a mutual working agreement where the details of the job, workload, and future of a job are related to the pay and compensation for the position.

 Conclusion: Both parties should be excited about the deal being done in a "win-win" situation. If either party is not, that spells trouble will arrive soon and both parties are then in a "lose-lose" situation.

4. The "Gunner Attitude"

"Just about everyone in business knows that physicians have a poor acumen for business."

We often celebrate in medicine the student who seems to know everything. The gunner wants to come across as being very impressive to more senior staff and faculty. Sometimes they come off as being obnoxious and overbearing with a flair of one-upping their peers in an attempt to support their own glory. They are quick to raise their hands in grade school and seem to always have the correct answer to impress their teachers. When working on rounds in the hospital as a medical student, they always seem to have read well ahead of what has been covered in class. If they ask a question, it will often be profound and thought provoking, and they will essentially answer it themselves in order to amaze.

 Mistake: Thinking that because you know medicine, you know business.

All physicians have been celebrated academically at some point, if not most points, throughout their academic careers. As leaders of the treatment team and the perceived heads of the medical hierarchy, we can be held in both earned and unearned reverence. Much of this makes sense with the time and dedication that we have given to our academics and dedication to our field. As physicians, we are trained to attempt to know as much as possible regarding a given disease state. At the same time, there are multiple variables to every patient. Much of medicine is not hard science like mathematics and physics. But we are trained that given a specific set of facts, algorithms, and statistics, we can make an educated guess. In the medical hierarchy, we are the most trained at guessing.

The issue is that we often take this behavior and accolades into the business world, of which we have had little or no training. Just about everyone in business knows that physicians have a poor acumen for business. Everyone seems to know this except for physicians. We are trained to believe in our educated guesses, even if the foundations of our facts are scarce at best. The problem in contracts and business is that there are others who have a lot more knowledge and experience. I'm not saying that a doctor cannot know business, but if the doctor does know, it was not taught in the standard medical curriculum. In these matters, our education can fail us. The problem is that due to many of our gunner attitudes, we are the last to know, and when many of us do know, it is well too late.

Oftentimes this gunner attitude that is celebrated by some in medicine leads us to believe that the physician should know everything and be the first to speak out to show it. It gives the idea that if you do not know, then obviously you are weak, a poor study, and not as smart as the rest of us. With this gunner attitude, we fail to realize that asking questions helps to grow our understanding. I remember my father, who was a computer analyst, once saying that "if I speak too quickly, then everyone will know what I know and what I don't, but if I stay silent, I have what I know and gain what they know, as well." As President Abraham Lincoln said, "Better to remain silent and be thought a fool than speak out and remove all doubt." Remember that being silent is to gain information and speaking to ask questions only begets growth of knowledge. Unlike much of our training in medicine, asking questions shows a potential employee's interest, not ignorance.

Don't Be Quick to Make Your Argument

It is important to make sure you have knowledge of your needs and/
or the job's needs before making your argument for demands. In our
"gunner" spirit, we can be quick to speak and slow to listen. Many
times we can talk ourselves right out of a good deal when we fail to
listen because we act as if we know business as much as we know
medicine.

Business Knows That Doctors Don't Know

As doctors we often believe that we know business because we are
very smart. In order to become a doctor, you have to be smart. We
are all essentially smart academically and in the science of medicine.
Many times this causes us to believe that this knowledge of medicine
transitions to the business side of medicine. The issue is that the
ignorance of the business often causes us to not even know what
we don't know. It is possible to be running a race where you are so
far behind that you actually believe you are ahead. It would be like
running the track at the Olympics, and as you lean forward to nip
the leading competitor at the finish line, you soon find that you have
another lap to go. I truly believe that our training leaves us that igno-
rant about how the business side of medicine works.

Always Ask Questions

It is important to always ask questions. I would go further to say
always ask questions whether you know the answer or not. The reason to do this is not to be disingenuous, but to gauge the knowledge
of the people you are talking to, as well as to see how honest and
truthful they are. If you hear an all-out fable of the truth, then make
sure you are very careful about your further interactions. Pay close
attention to a liar. If a person is lying or misleading before you sign
a contract, you can expect it will only get worse after you sign on
the dotted line. As will be covered later, remember that contracts are
only as good as the people you are signing with. The fight to get out
of a bad situation can be costly with your finances and your time.

Listen

Listening is a key in any contract negotiation. One would expect that physicians are great listeners due to patient care and the need to elicit symptoms from patients we serve. In the case of fast-paced twenty-first-century medicine where caseloads are high, but time is short, it has been shown that doctors' listening skills are very poor. It is important to listen to a potential employer's needs. Listening to their needs will give potential clues on how you may meet those needs. Do not base your options on assumptions. You are more able to meet those needs and see where you fit with multiple options. It is important that you get as much history as possible, but in getting that history, it is important to understand what their needs are.

> **Conclusion:** Listen first in order to have effective negotiation. You give yourself an opportunity to learn when you listen. Speaking too quickly will definitely give an advantage to the other negotiator simply because they are learning more than you.

5. Where Are You in Your Job Search and Professional Career?

I often hear statements from doctors who are no longer in residency and are out practicing stating that contract negotiations are for doctors coming out of residency, but since they are established and out working, they do not need this information. They fail to realize how important this is and how doctors sign or resign contracts their entire working career.

Example

> I remember seeing a classmate of mine at a convention. I told him that I was about to do a talk on contract negotiations, and he stated to me that it sounds to be an interesting topic that a lot of doctors don't know but need to know more about. I invited him to the session, and his response was that because he worked mostly locum tenens jobs, he did not need to know information on negotiating a contract.

 Mistake: Taking what seems to be a great job that does not fit with where you are in your career.

Dr. False Start

Where you are in life clearly determines the type of job that you are looking for. A resident is looking for a job that will use their skill and pay well. For the most part, they are eager to work, young, vibrant, energetic, and want to make as much money as possible. Much of this is due to needing to pay back undergraduate and medical school loans, desiring to live the life of their other professional friends who have homes and nice cars, and desiring to catch up on all the delayed gratification from spending twelve to sixteen years in education past high school. This type of doctor often makes mistakes in picking their first job, due to not clearly knowing the type of work they are getting into and due to a lack of on-the-job experiences.

Dr. Grant Hussle

Other times, you may be on your "grind or hustle" where you are looking forward to making as much legitimate money as possible and going for the highest bidder of services. This is the doctor who is negotiating for the highest dollar. Typically, they don't stay in one place long because if someone offers "another nickel over lunch money," they are quickly out the door. They are normally nomadic in nature and do not often make friends where they are or unpack their luggage. Also, this person may have a steady job, but is willing to do extra call, work on weekends, or cover for others in order to increase their income. The contract they are looking for is the dollar with efficiency.

Dr. Ness Egg

Frequently, a late-career physician may be looking to decrease hours, move to an area where they can retire, and maximize benefits that will help them build a comfortable nest egg. Many government or large corporation jobs fit the bill for these people, due to retirement packages and the work being fairly consistent from day to day. Many physicians are attempting to take full advantage of matching funds and are looking for the location to retire.

Dr. E.Z. St. Eddy

Around mid-career, a lot of physicians determine that they are in a lot of debt after living it up those first few years of independent practice outside of residency. At this time, work is no longer a novelty; you have the rhythm of your profession and career. You are still eager to move forward in your profession, but there is a practicality to what you are doing as well. Some of us may hit our comfort zone by then and will hit an easy and steady work rhythm. It would be great if we were working in a job that we find to be our right fit for the rest of our lives, or we may find that this job just isn't it, but we have a better idea of what we are looking for. They are the "I've got a job; I just want a better one" type.

Dr. Ned Job Asap

This group is the physicians who are either trying to get out of a bad situation where they don't like where they are or possibly they had some trouble along the way. Many times you find these people running to something due to having to run away from something else. Oddly enough, the last problem catches up and shows quickly at the next job opportunity. Sometimes there has been an unexpected move, a falling out at the last job, or a change in life. Sometimes a doctor may just be out of work and needs to get back in the job market. These doctors are looking for the first contract that makes sense to take.

 Conclusion: You must know where you are in your career before taking a job. Sometimes a great opportunity may have poor timing.

II.

Friends with Benefits

6. Benefit Packages

Benefit packages are pre-tax funds that come out of your paycheck before you receive it. Remember that as a doctor, you are in the middle to upper-middle class of income. This means that in the United States, you share the burden of paying essentially the highest tax rate. Every dime you can save is to your benefit.

 Mistake: Taking the lowest premium and believing this will save your out-of-pocket cost.

The benefit package can make or break the desirability of a job, and it is a very important part of an employee's salary. I remember getting my first job as a twenty-five-year-old resident physician and attending a full day or two of employee orientations, seminars, and lectures on everything from sexual harassment, fires, bomb threats, hurricane evacuations, 401(k) options, and the different benefit plans available. I found myself quite bored with the employee information seminars. As I sat there, it was difficult to pay attention and hard to keep from nodding off. Although I was not present in my department at the time, I still didn't want to look like a slacker on my first official day on the job by sleeping through employee orientation. Being young at the time and not well versed on employee benefits packages, I found myself struggling to understand the information presented, and looking back I see that I did not clearly know the relevance in what all was going on. A person got up in front of a group of at least fifty of us, ran through information, and then asked us to select an option from health care, vision, dental, 401(k) options, state retirement plan, and picking between low- to high-risk mutual funds.

Health Benefits

"It is important to know that when the employer is negotiating rates, for the most part, the employer's concern is the best rate for the employer and not the employee."

Health Maintenance Organizations (HMOs)

A Health Maintenance Organization (HMO) is health insurance that has a set of physicians whose services are contracted with. Most HMOs have a fairly large number of network providers. In an HMO, the employee is required to have a primary care doctor who manages their overall health. If more specialty care is required, then he will refer you to another physician within your HMO. If you are seeing a physician outside of the HMO, your health insurance may not cover the visit or the treatment because it was done outside of the network of physicians within the HMO.

Preferred-Provider Organizations (PPOs)

Preferred Provider Organizations allow more flexibility when choosing a physician. The monthly premium costs tend to be higher than with Health Maintenance Organizations, but you have more options. Some services may not be covered and there can be more out-of-pocket costs.

High-Deductible Health Plans

Many individuals and employers are choosing to go with high-deductible health plans. This type of plan helps if you are a healthy person and don't expect to be ill or you are willing to pay out of pocket for things that are not expensive. This type of plan allows security that, if a costly medical issue arises, you will have insurance to help with the costs. I have seen these deductibles as low as $500 or as high as $5,000. Patients who choose this option and have a deductible of $5,000 are essentially cash pay patients unless they are going to be hospitalized or are going to require an expensive procedure. The monthly deductible is typically the lowest. The high-deductible health plans are often used along with Medical Saving Accounts. An individual would place pre-taxed monies into a medical savings account and then would spend the money from the account for health care costs. This account would earn interest and be able to roll to another investment account. You can withdraw the funds from the account. There are rules on the amount of deposits and on how the funds may be withdrawn.

Remember, employers may cover health plans differently. Some employers pay 100 percent of the premium, some pay 50 percent, and some pay 0 percent. If the employer pays 0 percent of the premium, then you are essentially self-insured. Typically, large employers will be able to negotiate better rates from insurance companies because the volume of employees and potential patients give bargaining power. It is important to know that when the employer is negotiating rates, for the most part, the employer's concern is the best rate for the employer and not the employee. There is no guarantee that the employer's health insurance program is better than an individual shopping for insurance.

Vacation and Sick Leave

There can be a lot of variability with how this is done. Most common is a two-week paid vacation where the employee gives advance notice of the leave. Sick leave may be another ten to fourteen days per year. Other leaves are maternity, paternity, professional development and protective time, family medical leave, unscheduled leaves, and mental health leave, to mention a few.

As you can see, all these different leaves add up, especially if they are all paid leave. Professional development may be anywhere from

$250 and two days per year to any amount of money and time. This means a lot if you are given funds for professional development and the company is footing the bill for medical conference in Australia (er, cough . . . two-week vacation).

Expenses and Expense Accounts

Another important aspect to remember is the cost of expenses. Just about every professional requires a cell phone, and many of us require to be connected to the web twenty-four hours per day. Are you able to expense that through your company? If your cell phone/communication bill runs $200 per month and the company fully reimburses you for that, then you are making another $2,400 per year. Do they require you to have a smartphone, tablet, or the like? Do they pay the expenses for it? If so, your overall income is actually higher if the company is paying for this.

If you work in an urban area where parking can be scarce, the cost of parking a car can be tremendous. Even if it is $5 per day, you have to multiply and it becomes a $1,200 yearly expense. I know in some urban areas it can easily be $25 per day or higher to park. Whether you park a car or not, you have to keep in mind the time to travel to the job. I consider travel a part of the workday. If it takes an hour to and an hour from a job, then the workday is increased by two hours every day. Gas, tolls, and tokens all add up in money and the stress of a commute. To some it may not seem much and just a part of working, but this definitely wears you mentally and costs financially over time.

 Conclusion: Make sure your benefit package fits your and your family's individual needs. You must consider your career, finances, and health and your dependents as well. Make sure you select wisely. The benefit package can truly make or break a negotiation

7. Salary Versus Independent Contractor

Work Duties

It is important to understand how compensation is set up. Are you being hired into a salary position or as an independent contractor? You may determine this by looking at the terms and conditions of employment. An independent contractor is a person who works for themselves in that they are their own boss, but at the same time, they are contracting their services to another entity or business. An employee works at the direction of the employer. One is contracting their services to do a specific job while the other is directed to do a job at the direction of the employer.

 Mistake: Not purchasing your own disability, life, or medical insurance as an independent contractor.

 Mistake: Assuming that because you work for a big company, the employee's interest is first when the company gives options for a disability, life, and medical insurance packages.

Example

An independent contracting physician who has their own private practice may work at a local emergency room for a specific number of hours. This person essentially has their own practice, but is doing work outside of their practice. A salaried employee would be a person who is an employee of the hospital and is directed by the hospital itself to work in the ER.

Example

A doctor is an outpatient clinician employee for West Side General Hospital. He can only treat patients at West Side's outpatient clinic. He then admits patients to West Side General Hospital. He is not allowed to work for East Side as a hospitalist. It would be a conflict of interest for West Side to pay him as a salaried employee in their outpatient clinic if he were to admit patients for himself to treat at East Side. The conflict in interest is that West Side would be losing patients to East Side. An independent contractor, on the other hand, could work at West Side Hospital two days per week, but at the same time work weekends as a hospitalist at East Side. The contractor who can work both places is neither an employee of West or East Side.

Compensation

HOURLY, DAILY, PER PATIENT, PER COLLECTIONS, OR YEARLY SALARY

Are you being paid hourly, daily, per patient, per collections, or are you on a yearly salary? If the daily rate is $1,000 for an eight-hour day, then the equivalent hourly rate is $125 per hour. If the going rate for a paid physician is an estimated $125 per hour and another job offers payment by the *individual patient* seen, then that equivalent by the patient job would be about $35 per patient if it is estimated that you would see three to four patients per hour. *Per collection* is similar to being paid per patient except that how much you make will be directly correlated to the ability to bill and collect. If the place has a lot of low-income non-insured patients, then this would not be optimum. The opposite is optimum if the office is mostly cash and has a population that has the ability and is willing to pay. For yearly salaries, it is assumed that there will be a benefits package included.

So although a salaried position will on average pay less than an hourly or daily rate, this is made up in the benefits package. The benefits package can be worth on average another 20 to 30 percent above the salary.

Tax Rates

"If a person is an independent contractor, then the contractor must pay their own taxes."

The difference is particularly important in paying taxes. If a person is an employee, the employer must deduct payroll taxes and social security from the employee. If a person is an independent contractor, then the contractor must pay their own taxes. An employee is assumed to only be able to work for the employer.

Salaried Benefit Packages

"It is important that an independent contractor shops for policies that tailor to them."

Also, an employee is typically tied into benefits, while an independent contractor is not. If a doctor is receiving medical benefits, paid vacation, sick days, and a retirement plan, then they are most likely an employee. Most often an independent contractor would not be receiving these options. So typically an independent contractor will receive more money on an hour-to-hour basis than an employee, but this is a substituted loss for not receiving benefits. It would be expected that a physician, who is an independent contractor, would have their own benefits set up.

A side note: I would recommend that all independent contractors have life insurance if they have a family or spouse who depends on their income. More importantly, the independent contractor needs disability insurance along with medical insurance.

Remember that employees have the benefit of being under a large group, so many times their insurance is negotiated by the large company for a lower rate. At the same time, realize that the rates are negotiated by the company with the company's best interest in mind. The insurance policies may not be the best for the individual employee. Some salaried employees may even want to have additional benefits that they are paying independent of the company they are working for. It is important that an independent contractor shops for policies that tailor to them. The prices can be very different between insurance companies, so make sure you do your research. The advantage of the individual is that the plan is specific to your needs and not the needs of the company or group.

 Conclusion: With either salaried or contracted employment, it is important to understand your tax situation and have benefits. Trust me when I say pay your taxes. It is partly the inspiration for this book.

III.

Compensation and Money

8. What about the Money?

What Am I Worth?

For the most part, physicians do not know their value in the marketplace. If you are ever admitted to a hospital or visit an emergency room, you will typically get two bills. One bill is from the hospital and the other is from the physician. There is a difference between the amounts of the bills. For a one-night stay, the hospital services bill may be $3,000 and the physician service bill may be $250. Often it is a fraction of the hospital bill.

 Mistake: Not realizing the value of a physician.

What many physicians do not realize is that the hospital cannot bill until the physician or the medical extender sees the patient. It is similar to how baseball works. Nothing happens until the pitcher throws the ball. There is no game of baseball if the pitcher does not throw the ball. The pitcher is the catalyst of the entire game. That is one of the reasons why the pitching staff is central to any major league baseball team and pitchers are often the highest paid players. Unlike baseball, where pitchers salaries go up, doctor salaries are going down. *The fact is that a person who throws a 98-mile-per-hour*

fastball, an off-speed pitch with good movement, and a wicked curve ball is more valuable than a pediatric trauma surgeon saving lives night in and night out. These examples are to show that nothing is billed in medicine until the physicians sees the patient, writes the clinical note, and signs that the patient has been seen. This is very valuable and powerful, and many physicians have lost sight of that.

When Do I Ask about Money?

Typically it is the employer's responsibility to bring up compensation for work. I would say that it is most common that people seeking employment first want to know how much will they be paid. People will want a number even before they know exactly what the job entails. I once met a person who stated that it would take at least $300,000 before he would even consider a job. I questioned the demand because the current market value for the job did not justify that amount. Also, depending on the expectations of the job, the amount you may be asking for could possibly be under what you should be paid. This, of course, depends on the actual job.

Realize that you almost never want to tell an employer the lowest you will take, especially at the beginning of a negotiation. The amount you give will often be the maximum that is offered, and a potential employer's negotiator, who is looking to save the employer money, may try to step you down from that amount. Although it was your intent to give the minimum you would take, you also may have sealed in the maximum that you will be offered. I've also seen those who will lowball themselves, thinking that they are getting ahead and hoping to ensure that they will get the job.

The other issue is that the job may seem as if it is overpaying you, but pay close attention to the amount of work or stress that is required. If after doing your homework on a particular salary the job is offering more than expected, then take a careful look to see if something is missing. As the adage goes, if something sounds too good to be true, then it probably is.

Example

I once had a good friend who took a job working at a medium-sized local hospital where she was the lone physician covering an ICU. I had been working in the hospital and always saw this one physician covering, and so I made the statement that it seemed as if she lived there. She assured me that she did not. I stated to her that it seemed as if any time I walked on the floor, she was always there. She said that she was the only physician covering the ICU and that the hospital had been looking for over a year for someone else to hire full time in order to give her relief. The current relief that she had was four days a month by a contracting physician doctor who would do twenty-four-hour shifts. She was able to spend many nights at home. This was suitable because she lived in a high rise only a few blocks from the hospital. But depending on the acuity of the ICU, she also stayed many nights at the hospital. She felt well compensated for the work she did. Of course there was a question regarding the rights of a worker and that doctors have rights as well, but she felt that the hospital was really trying their best to get additional help and believed it would be coming soon. I asked myself why the hospital would be in any rush to find her help when they are getting two docs for the price of one and a quarter. At eighteen months into the job, she was still waiting on the help to come.

You frequently find that it is the immature negotiator who wants to know the salary before they know the job. In all actuality, you should know the salary before you even go to interview for the job. You know this information by doing your homework and research regarding how much the job pays. Much of this can be simply done online. Some websites that are helpful are www.careerbuilder.com and www.salary.com. Also, for most public universities, you can go online and look up how much the individual physicians are compensated. So, if you are looking at a potential academic nephrologist in St. Louis, Missouri, simply do a search for the salary of a "St. Louis

+ nephrologist + academia." This should give a roundabout idea of what you should expect to make.

When potential employees ask for high-dollar amounts, they often don't realize that the employer is making somewhat of a gamble that you will be able to help turn profit for the business, school, or department. If you are new and without any additional job skills above people who are working there, then it is hard for a person to explain why they are worth more than employees who have been there for years and may have more experience than the person requesting a higher salary.

Now I definitely "overstand" the thought of if you don't ask, you won't receive. Or the adage of "quiet mouths don't get fed." But you should know the approximate amount of what will be offered. Sometimes people do not know that they are being offered a very good and competitive compensation. The problem is that they may not realize the deal they have been given and may not take advantage. Or they may be asking for further negotiations regarding an increase in pay and do not grasp that they already have the advantage in pay. This can upset a potential employer because the person may not feel you are appreciative of the offer, or they quickly start to consider other people they can get for the same or lesser amount that may be more skilled. They are more than likely to have multiple options if they are paying more than the market value for the area.

What if the Pay Is Lower than Expected?

"You want the discussion to be based on facts."

It is not uncommon to face a situation where the pay does not seem to be what would be expected for the work. Make sure that you have done your homework and review if you missed something. If you are interested in the job and the offer is lower than projected, it is fair and expected that you should ask for what you believe the offer should be. Try to get better clarification on the difference between what is expected and what is being offered. If the potential employer stands by the offer, then it is best to justify your position with hard numbers. You want to avoid an opinionated discussion about why you deserve more. You want the discussion to be based on facts.

Example

> It's like buying a used car. Let's say the sticker price on the 2011 import car on the lot is $40,000, but the Kelley Blue Book suggested retail price is $36,000. It is listed on their website for $34,000. If they are sticking with the $40,000, or suggest any price that is more than the web price without justification, then it is suggested that you move on. Other dealers are more than willing to sell you the same year, make, and model. Likewise, appreciate that there are other people offering jobs, as well.

Make sure that your numbers are based on specifics of the job market. Show the potential employer what your facts are based upon and have them explain why they are not correct. Many times it can be a misunderstanding that is simple to explain. The listed offer might be old, the job may actually be different than what was stated, the company may have gone through changes, or it could be a misstatement of information.

You want to clarify any ambiguity or uncertainty. This is often done when you feel the job description is underpaying for the responsibilities of the job. Many times during negotiations, it is possible to walk away due to a deal not being fairly compensated. Either of these two will cause an uncomfortable work environment. Even though most employers are looking to give a fair compensation for a doctor, there are some that are not.

If you notice that the compensation has a large disparity from the workload, it is important to ask the question "Why?" If you do mention this, then you should have information to explain why you believe so.

The other side of this is when we believe we are getting ahead if we are compensated above value. If you see this, then be a bit wary of the large discrepancy. It is not common for an employer to overpay for an employee. This is true even if the employee is a physician. It may be that a person has misunderstood the scope of the work. It is important to remember that in most businesses, including medicine, the profit margin is small. If a company is overpaying people and not bringing in income to support, then this is not a strong company. Realize that once they determine that you are overpaid, they may begin looking for someone to pay at the correct value, ultimately leaving you without a job.

Negotiate the Next Contract

Remember that your value is always reassessed. If you are ever going to negotiate for a higher salary or look for a higher position of employment in a company, then you need to make sure you are doing your current job correctly. It is difficult to argue the point of deserving a pay increase when you are a poorly effective employee. Also realize that your performance on the job may help keep you from losing your job. Understand that all jobs go through ups and downs. There are times of multiple hires and also layoffs. It is rare for a company to be around for more than ten years, so it is understandable that your job may not last forever. People will remember the type of work you put in at a previous location and will remember you for the next position. The reason that some doctors always seem to get the best opportunities is because they do well in the current opportunity.

 Conclusion: Understand your value as a physician. Research the job market in the area and the salaries or your specialty doing similar work.

9. Key Factors Other than Money

Many times people will make their ultimate decision on whether or not to take a job based upon money. This is a flawed approach and possibly a fatal mistake. Of course compensation is very important, but there are other factors that you have to be aware of.

 Mistake: Assuming an opportunity is great based on salary alone.

Time

It is also important to consider the time that is involved. Understand that time can be difficult to figure out from a job description in that a forty-hour workweek job is more than forty hours when you add in unexpected late days and call schedules.

Example

Northside Hospital pays $200,000 per year and requires a forty-hour workweek with no call or weekends. Southside Hospital pays $250,000 per year for a forty-hour workweek, but in addition it requires every third night telephone call coverage and one weekend per month onsite hospital call. All of a sudden the forty-hour workweek of the $250,000 job is a sixty-hour-a-week job. In comparison, the former makes more money per hour with all nights and weekends free, while the latter makes more per week, but has to lose nights and weekends and overall makes less money per hour.

Volume of Patients

It is imperative to know the volume of patients that you will be taking care of in the run of a day. How many patients you are seeing should have a direct effect on the amount you expect to be compensated for.

Example

Let's use the example of $200,000 per year versus $250,000 per year again. Northside Hospital pays $200,000 per year and the doctor is scheduled to see twenty to twenty-five patients per day, while the Southside Hospital is paying $250,000 for the doctor to see forty-five to fifty patients per day. The $200,000 doctor is making more money per patient and has a lower stress level and carries a lower volume of patients than the $250,000 doctor. This lower volume translates to less paper work, managing fewer consumers, less fatigue, and a lower risk of burnout over time.

Intensity

You have to look at the location where you will work. Some work areas are more time consuming and have a higher level of acuity than others. Managing a ten-bed ICU most often will be a lot more demanding than managing a twenty-hospital-bed floor. Managing a twenty-person-per-day outpatient clinic can be different than seeing twenty patients in a hospital. The important point to remember is the intensity of the day greatly depends on the location that you are working in.

Location and Support Staff

This can make or break a work environment. I remember working at a large urban university hospital where there were a lot of supporting staff, including nurse practitioners, RNs, LVNs, CNAs, and other ancillary services, such as respiratory techs all the way to orderlies who were helping transport patients. Also, the hospital had multiple residency programs and medical students. The work as the attending physician was fairly simple and was essentially a supervisory position. This can be very different than working in a small rural hospital that does not have the support staff and ancillary services of a large institution. So, even though the volume of patients is a lot less, the amount of work is a lot more due to having to do multiple patient care services without the support staff. Next thing you know, you are calling families, calling hospitals, and covering the ER, ICU, and another doctor's service while being the only physician on site.

 Conclusion: Understand that there is more value to a job than the salary itself. It is easy to make the mistake that the job is great because it pays well. Possibly even more important is time required, volume of patients, and support staff. There is a lot more to value in a job than money.

10. Knowledge Is Power

If you want the upper hand in a negotiation, your most powerful tool is knowledge. It is important to educate yourself as much as possible about your potential employer. You get a lot of this from the job description.

 Mistake: Not bothering to research the job, the area, and location and how it will affect your lifestyle and family.

Example

BOARD-CERTIFIED MD

SUBURBAN OUTPATIENT PRACTICE

2 SATELLITE LOCATIONS

SHARED CALL WITH 2 PHYSICIANS

MUST LIVE WITHIN 30 MINUTES
OF LOCAL HOSPITAL

Suburban outpatient practice with shared call of two physicians and having to live within thirty minutes of the hospital gives a strong hint that you are going to be busy and every third night you will be hinged to the hospital. For an obstetrician or intensive, this may be protocol for many. This description would be odd for a dermatologist.

Location and Region

You want to research the location. With the example above, you clearly want to know about the suburb. Remember to ask, if you are considering taking this job, what the area is like. You can go online to the local chamber of commerce to look at medium incomes, age demographics, services, museums, parks, climate, and seasons. With my family living and growing up in Houston, we considered doing residency up north. My wife clearly told me that she was not living anywhere north after living in Nashville, Tennessee, and going through a cold front where it was five degrees outside with a wind chill of negative twenty. This would be a harsh arctic blast for people living in the northern United States, and for native Houstonians, this is considered cruel and unusual punishment.

If you are single, it may be less desirable to live in a suburban area if you do not have quick access to a city. If you are married with children, then it is important to know what the school system is like and what the work opportunities are for your spouse. Depending on your spouse's career, the location may not work for the family if the spouse must put their life on hold for you to have the job you want. There are too many jobs to take one where you know your spouse will be unhappy before you start.

Volume

It is important to know what type of volume a particular clinic does. Is this a high-volume clinic? Is the suburb growing or losing population? If it is a slow clinic, but is in a growing area, then your prospects look great, but do you have time to wait on the changing demographics? Are the other two physicians' schedules full? If not, then why are they hiring? Are there physician extenders? How many patients are the extenders seeing? If they don't have the volume, are you paid by the patient contact, by the hour, or in a salaried position? What is the patient volume of the satellite clinics? Where are they located? What is the distance of the satellite clinic to the hospital and to your home? Where do you admit the patients at the satellite clinic? Are you admitting them to the hospital nearest to the satellite office and do you cover inpatients at the other hospital, or is there another service that follows the patients at the second hospital?

Time

Know how much time they need from you. Most job descriptions will say "forty-hour workweek." Most physician jobs are not forty-hour workweeks. It is important to know how many patients you will be seeing a week. If, for example, it says twenty patients per day, then you need to know twenty of what kind of patients. Twenty outpatients in a day are different than twenty inpatients per day. Are the twenty outpatients all follow-ups, new evaluations, or a combination? Are they inpatients on a medical/surgical floor; are there any patients in the ICU; are you covering admissions; are there residents, medical students, physician extenders, etc.? If you are doing outpatient and inpatient, are the consults during the middle of your rounds or during the middle of a busy clinic? Consults and trips to the ER during the middle of a busy clinic or inpatient service can disrupt the entire day, cause for poor patient satisfaction if they are waiting on you and cause your day to be very haphazard with not knowing if you will finish at five p.m. or nine p.m. The lack of knowing when you are headed home causes a lot of stress due to the unpredictability of your schedule.

 Conclusion: When considering a job, make sure you research the type of work and workload beforehand. Researching the job is extremely important, but also as important is the impact of the region, location, and lifestyle and your career goals and your family.

IV.

CLOSING THE DEAL

11. The Interview (Game-Day Preparations)

"People love to hear about themselves, and it is impressive that you took the time to look them up."

Research the People

Make sure you review the website for the company or business and know the basics, such as the organizational structure and hierarchy. Know the strengths and weaknesses of where you are interviewing. Research the people you are talking to, if you know who they are before the interview. People love to hear about themselves, and it is impressive that you took the time to look them up. There are things that people will expect for you to know before the interview, such as who is the owner or chairperson. Look up the type of work they do and in what the company or persons you are interviewing with specialize. The Internet has a ton of information regarding professionals. It is a turnoff to see someone who is unprepared.

 Mistake: Not prepping yourself for the interview.

Who Are You Talking To?

It is important to know whom you are negotiating with. Is this the person who makes the final decision, or do they give suggestion to who makes the final decision? Many times we think that we want to talk directly to "The Man" (or the woman) when making decisions on employment because if we could talk to him, then we could impress the person in charge. Well, that is not always the case. The person in charge may have a lot of responsibilities, and it is fairly safe to trust that their designated person is the one you need to impress. It is important to realize that hiring the right person is vital to any company and this is taken very seriously. If the person in front of you is not the primary person who makes decisions, that is just fine. If you can impress that person, you have a pretty good chance of getting the job.

I've seen some cases where a person will dismiss the interviewer if that person does not make the final decision. This is a grave mistake. Many times that person is the one who makes the decision solely because their recommendation directly influences the boss. Realize that the boss is going to be a very busy person and may not have the chance to review all hires. Also remember that everyone in the office is interviewing you, as well. That includes the front desk clerk and everyone else who knows that you may be potentially working there. I've done interviews where the person seemed to be a good person, but it was clear that they did not fit the office environment and may have difficulty on the job. Now this does not mean the person would not be hired, but it does bring cause for concern for office milieu.

Your Dress

An interviewer will see how you look in your interview clothes, how you feel in your touch (handshake), and how you sound in your communication. All people make snap judgments in evaluating others, especially when they are there specifically to evaluate you. They are trying or even being paid to make these decisions quickly. It is safe to assume that you met the criteria for the job when they invited you to be interviewed. They brought you in for them and you to have a closer look. That first look starts with how you are dressed. In dress, I recommend to always be professional.

Example

I remember once seeing a person interview for a job they were sure they were going to receive. They had previously worked there, but had left for a couple of years for another opportunity. They knew all the interviewers as colleagues, the position needed to be filled, and the interviewee had the job skills to do the job well. The person arrived in a sundress and sandals and conducted themselves in a very casual manner to the point of bringing up office politics and even gossip at the interview. Subsequently, the shoo-in did not get the job.

It is best to be professional. It is better to be overdressed for an interview than to be underdressed. It is best to be conservative and businesslike in dress. When I was in medical school at Meharry Medical College, I remember the president, Dr. John Maupin, stating to the matriculating third years into clinical rotations, "It is great to be an individual, but no one is obligated to pay you for your individuality."

I recommend a business suit for both men and women. Make sure the suit is tailored to your body contour. No matter how expensive or "cute" a suit may be, if it does not fit correctly, then you and the suit look cheap. A coat and tie for men and a business suit for women. A job for a physician may not require a formal suit, but at least be business professional. The grunge look went out in the nineties and the "sexy and I know it" look went out soon thereafter. It is not the right time to show skin in an interview. Granted, you may have great "assets," but you don't want to get a job based on this. To employers, it looks unprofessional, and you don't want to accentuate that you are not serious about the job and will become a distraction in the workplace.

Another note for women: I recommend that a woman wear comfortable heels because you do not know how long you will have to be standing. It is not cute to take off your heels in an interview setting. Even though stilettos and tall platforms may be appealing, they do not feel appealing after standing for extended periods of time.

I feel most comfortable when I'm dressed well and look nice. I wouldn't recommend being too flashy, but looking nice is never a bad thing. The opposite is true. Looking bad is a bad thing. Some would say that you should not look too nice because you don't want what you are wearing to outshine or steal the show from what you are conveying as a potential employee. Honestly, I have not met a suit that I saw a person put on that outshined the content of what they had to say, not unless the person had nothing to say.

What I would say about this is that often women are more apt to pay attention to detail and men are not. In today's society, most do not anticipate if the person is going to be a male or female. Women are more likely to notice if your suit, shirt, and tie do not match in color or style. Women will notice scruffy shoes that haven't been shined since eighth grade prom. Looking nice will impress people. Looking bad is not impressive, but also stepping in the door like a peacock is overkill. There is a difference between casual, business-casual, professional, formal, and party wear.

Handshake

Make sure you have a good handshake. Many times you can lose an interview from the handshake. You should look someone in the eye when shaking their hand because it gives a look of honesty, and looking off to the side shows disinterest or deceit. The hand should be firm to touch, but not too firm, which comes off as a bit odd, narcissistic, or controlling. It should not be a soft grab where your hand does not grip the other person's. At times, you will feel where women do not press palm to palm and they give a light grip with mostly fingers. When interviewing for a job, it is not to your advantage to display weakness with a weak grab. It is not advantageous to have a shake that is flirtatious with a palm down, extended, elevated arm, with a four-finger light grip. Cold, wet, clammy hands are uncomfortable to touch, as well. Of course, we cannot control our autonomics at times, but if your hand is sweaty, try to dry it off before the grip, and if they are cold, attempt to warm them up by lightly rubbing them together.

Communicate

Make sure that you clearly communicate your interest to the interviewer. You should not expect the interviewer to know the type of work environment and compensation you are looking for. Make sure there are things you want to communicate and have your talking points to sell yourself. Have your questions prepared when the information has not already been presented. Be clear in speech and project with a tone of confidence, but not arrogance.

Other Things

Do not arrive too early. It is good to get to the interview approximately ten minutes before the interview time. That does not mean that you cannot arrive at the building until that time, because you want to give yourself plenty of time for the unexpected and possibly settle your nerves before walking into the interview. Remember that everyone is busy and you may inconvenience the interviewer by arriving thirty minutes early, and then they feel the obligation to go ahead and start the interview, thereby increasing their angst. Obviously, disrupting someone's day and throwing off their schedule does not make for a favorable impression.

Remember that you are talking to people and you want to be pleasant to the senses. Make sure you lay off the onions. I love to "Eat Fresh," but be conscious of the scent of onions and bell peppers after eating lunch a couple of hours before. I don't care how much great information flows from your mouth, the interviewer will be distracted and may start to rush the interview just to get out of the room.

 Conclusion: It is important to make sure you are prepared for the day. Understand that by the time you have arrived for the interview, the employer is seriously interested and the interview is to seal the deal. Don't blow it due to a lack of preparation.

12. Media and the Fast New World of Negotiations

"Also, OMG, OMG, OMG, please do not have ridiculous pictures or statements on social media."

Be cautious in the brave new world of communication. There are a number of ways a potential employer may contact you. This may be over the phone, Internet, Facebook, Twitter, Google+, instant messaging, email, cell phones, text, and more. Even though this is not the preferred way to negotiate, it is convenient, but dangerous.

 Mistake: Not realizing that employers check your online statuses.

Many times when we are using these types of technology, we are easily distracted. It is not a good time to be discussing the direction of your professional career while driving in the morning rush-hour traffic or zooming down the freeway, weaving in and out of traffic at seventy miles per hour due to being late for work. To say the least, you are very distracted. Realize that the person you are negotiating with is not directly in front of you, so they have no idea what else is going on around you. It is often best to wait until you have time to be focused before negotiating. Likewise, it is not good to pick up the phone out of a dead sleep. You are typically at a disadvantage with a negotiation if you were not expecting a call from a potential employer due to an element of surprise and possibly being total-ly unprepared. I typically don't answer calls if I don't recognize the number, am not expecting the call, or it is not programmed into my smartphone. If it is important, they will leave a message.

Also, OMG, OMG, OMG, please do not have ridiculous pictures or statements on social media. Realize that employers check this stuff. If you allow me to friend you on your Facebook page or even Twitter, I can know exactly who you are. Your "friends" will let me know the type of person you are, your career, how you grew up, your interests, hobbies, sexual preference, and such.

Example

> **A human resource specialist posted pictures to her Face-book page during her cruise in the Caribbean. I would assume, to her, they seemed innocent enough, but taking pictures with drinks in your hands on a yacht with friends is not something you necessarily want your colleagues to see. Everyone seemed to notice the Instagram pic of her in her two-piece, one hand on hip, one hand holding a two-foot-long margarita, looking back at the camera with an accentuating booty pic. Upon returning from the cruise, it was obvious that she had not considered that half of her work team were also Facebook friends.**

Understand that private investigators are hired by large companies and firms to investigate potential clients and future employees. The first place to look is social media. Be careful what you put on social media. You do not know who is watching and who potentially will want to look.

 Conclusion: You social media presence is very important to employers and tells them a lot about you. If you feel that your social media presence is not you or could be embarrassing, then you need to change it.

13. Gut Feelings and Instincts

"If you see smoke, it serves to have caution before running into a burning building."

Remember to trust your "gut feelings" and intuition before making a deal. Your intuition mostly represents unconscious thoughts that are culminations of experience and knowledge gathered from bits and pieces of life experiences. When going into a good deal, there should be a level of excitement of the opportunity and a desire to get to work. It is most important to pay particular attention if the gut feeling gives you a "sick feeling" in your abdomen. This means something about what is going on does not feel right. It is kind of like walking in a dark parking lot and seeing a person wandering near your car. You are at a disadvantage because you are not able to see them well. They know that your intention is to get to your car, but you don't know exactly what their intention may be. Many times we will attempt to override our gut feeling and decide to walk to our car anyway. The same is true when going into a contract negotiation. If you feel you are walking into a dark parking lot, not sure of what is going to happen and feeling uneasy about the deal, then consider the consequences and make sure you have as much information as possible.

 Mistake: Not trusting yourself when you know something seems to be wrong.

I recommend not striking a deal if you feel uneasy. I would not just walk away, but it sounds as if there are some clarifications that need to be done. It may be good to speak to someone impartial about the company. Ask to speak to some of the other doctors who work for them and to those who have in the past. I've seen companies give references to physicians who have worked there previously who are open and honest in one way or another. Remember: where there is smoke, there is fire. If you see smoke, it serves to have caution before running into a burning building.

Get Factual Information

"It is key to bring unconscious fear to conscious reasoning."

If you have this gut feeling, then it is important to get more factual information. It is key to bring unconscious fear to conscious reasoning. If you are not sure about a deal one way or another and you find it worth figuring out, it is important that you do more homework and ask more questions. Other people who are knowledgeable are the secretaries and staff who work there. They may definitely have the inside scoop on the operations. You want to speak to the ancillary staff if you are able.

Cliques, Gangs, Thugs, and the Down-right Spooky

As I travel from early career physician to mid-career, I've seen some things in medicine. As the saying goes, "I may have been born yesterday, but I stayed up all night." I learned that if you hear something go bump in the middle of the night, it is best to check it out. Oddly enough, there are shady characters in medicine. You want to make sure that you are in the correct environment.

If an employer is saying something that sounds too good to be true, then it probably is. For example, if a job would normally pay $200,000 for a year and someone offers $450,000 for half the work, then something or someone is up to no good. You should know before you walk into the interview about how much you should be paid. If the numbers do not add up, then you need to get clarification.

Be extremely careful of what you sign. Just as identity theft can occur in your personal life and finances, this also can occur in your practice of medicine. So much of our information is in multiple places, such as on websites, hospital systems, insurance companies, and other places of business. If the federal government sees you listed as the doctor in charge, medical director, or staff employee who signs off on billing, then it is difficult to prove that you had no idea fraud was occurring, especially if you signed off on it. Fraud is rampant in medicine. According to the Department of Health and Human Services and the Department of Justice's Health Care Fraud and Abuse Control Program Annual Report for Fiscal Year 2010, Medicare fraud alone costs the United States over an estimated 60 billion dollars per year. Some would estimate that it could be much more. If you consider fraud with Medicaid and private insurance, you have to realize that this number is staggering.

If you notice anything odd that cannot be explained regarding monetary practices, then be very cautious. If you know something is wrong, then leave and get far, far away. With the amount of money spent on health care, understand that a little bit becomes a lot of bit and any bit can land you in jail. Losing or restricting your license, along with the cost of professional and public embarrassment, makes it not worth it.

The Contract Is Only as Good as the People Who Sign It

It is quite easy to say what you are going to do, but it is more difficult to write it down. At the same time, it is easy to write something down and then not do what is written. I have found that many people may write a contract knowing that they have no intention of fulfilling the contract. Even in medicine, there are multiple shady characters and companies out there. That is why it is important to get background information on the company by other physicians and the surrounding community. It is important to not base all your information on hearsay, but if a place has had multiple disgruntled employees, be very wary of signing with them.

Understand that the legal fight to get out of a contract can be costly. When dealing with many large organizations, they may have a team of lawyers who are on payroll to fight for their side of an issue. As an individual, your money and time invested may be a bit more finite. So it is important to know not only what the agreement is, but the integrity of people whose signatures are on it, as well.

 Conclusion: Trust your instincts. If your instincts tell you that something is wrong, then investigate what exactly that is. If it is fixable, then fix it. If not, then walk away.

14. Close but Not There: Final Negotiation Details

"There are too many scenarios to mention on how to work out the final details, but it is important to brainstorm the different ideas and scenarios in order to find a viable option."

Many times we may be close to getting the contract done, but not quite there. This could be due to monetary reasons or other work-related issues. If you are a single parent who is living out of town without family, it could be difficult to do a job where the work hours do not permit the ability to take school-age children to school or they make arranging overnight call difficult. It is important to attempt reasoning on how to make this work out. Many times it may be that the hospital can arrange day care. Maybe a cut in salary and working part time may be sufficient or cutting a few hours from the weekday and adding on a few hours on Saturday. If a parent is divorced with small children, then it may be worth the attempt to arrange call to occur when the children are spending every other weekend with the other parent. There are too many scenarios to mention on how to work out the final details, but it is important to brainstorm the different ideas and scenarios in order to find a viable option.

 Mistake: Giving up on a near-great opportunity due to a detail that could have been worked out.

You want to make sure that everything is clear regarding your needs and the potential employer's needs. If there are any misunderstandings, then ask questions. Many times a deal may get stuck simply because each party's primary desires are not clearly understood. So make sure you clarify all of your primary goals and the points that need to be worked out in negotiation. Make sure your issues are clear and give some ideas on how to resolve them.

If there is a problem that needs to be worked out, it is definitely to your advantage to have some solutions versus relying on the other party to come up with something. Your idea is more than likely to be in your favor than theirs. Also, by being clear and honest, the potential employer is better able to help. If you don't have a good idea on how to work it out, remember another option is to brainstorm regarding multiple different options. If you can't figure this out alone, then it is worth it to brainstorm with the potential employer. It is good to make sure that there is an understanding that these are just options and not demands or contractual agreements. You do have to worry about letting the person know what you are willing to give up to make the deal happen, but if you are at a point where it is not going to get done if you all can't come up with something, then there is not much to lose.

Also, it is not a good idea to make threats or demands. I know, I know—on TV and movies, a person makes a demand and the other person either calls the bluff or blinks and caves in due to the sheer power of the leading role. This is not typically how it happens. When demands are made when there is a discrepancy in an understanding, typically people will get a bad taste in their mouths regarding an employee; this disrupts the negotiating process, may destroy the relationship, and most likely will end the negotiation with two bitter parties parting. If you are the employee and the potential employer makes demands at the end of a negotiating process that is in the order of "take this deal or else," then I would definitely consider the else part of the deal and walk. Realize that the negotiating process and how well it goes is a window in how a company operates and treats its employees.

If you feel as if certain questions you have are not being answered, it is okay to ask the question again or reframe the question. Sometimes the person may be dodging the question or may truly not understand exactly the answer you are looking for. Be cautious when people are purposely evasive.

Remember there is the good and bad to all work environments. This even occurs in the "utopia" of medicine. There is no perfect job or position. If you believe so, you just either went through an excellent interview and you haven't started working there or you are honeymooning.

Don't feel rushed into a job. It is okay to pause for a second and ask to get back to the potential employer. It is a good idea to discuss the issue with a mentor or a trusted colleague. Remember that impulsive decisions may turn into long-term consequences. If there are parts of the deal that you like, then let the employer know, but for the points of discussion that are difficult, it is as important or even more important to let the employer know that, as well. It may be good to solidify the things that are mutually agreed upon and then discuss the sticky points. The drawback to this is that many times even the agreed points may need to change when the sticky points are accounted for.

Best Alternative to a Negotiated Agreement (BATNA)

The Best Alternative to a Negotiated Agreement (BATNA) was developed by Harvard Researchers Roger Fisher and William Ury. BATNA refers to what your next best option is if your preferred agreement is not satisfactory or is not able to be reached. Remember that your best option is having more than one option. The other option may be to develop an agreement that is not all that was desired with the potential employer but will work, or it could be to consider an option with a different employer that will work, as well.

It is important to have more than one option for employment. As the saying goes, "Do not put all your eggs in one basket." If you must be in a particular city or area, then look for more than one place of employment in that area. Some people will feel as if they must work in academia, and if they have to be in a particular city and there is only one medical academic center located there, then you have essentially eliminated a multitude of employment options. If you go on enough interviews with different entities, you may find that you enjoy the opportunities at more than one place. Essentially, make sure that you have options for other places of employment. After exploring these options, you may never know; something may be appealing that you had not initially considered.

What if I Really Want the Job?

"Even if this seems to be the perfect job for you, you still need to negotiate the contract to fit your particular needs."

Many times a physician will buy into a thought that this is the perfect job for me. It is great if a doctor finds that one perfect job. The question is: Have you looked at what exactly the job entails? It is hard to believe that one particular job does not have another that is near its equivalent. I would recommend to never be sold on just one particular job at one particular place. Even if this seems to be the perfect job for you, you still need to negotiate the contract to fit your particular needs.

It is not smart to be all in on one particular job before you investigate it. I've heard graduating residents say that it would be perfect if they could get a job at University of Best Ever because it is perceived that the job will carry prestige and give them instant notoriety. People may take advantage of this all-in attitude and may not offer as much because they know that you have tipped your hand in letting them know you will accept essentially anything they offer.

What if They Are Too Big?

Often physicians will feel that you cannot negotiate with a large entity. This comes from a lack of knowledge of a physician's worth. Many of us do not realize our value in the medical marketplace. We will often feel that we are not important enough to a hospital or facility to ask for what we want. Remember, as I mentioned before, in the medical model, nothing occurs until the physician sees that patient. It is not until a patient contact is done that a hospital can bill or collect money. Also understand that what the hospital collects has a lot more to do with ancillary services other than the physician's direct contact with patients. We forget about ordering lab work, imaging, and admissions. We fail to realize that the physician only keeps a small fraction of what they are generating for a company and the American economy.

 Conclusion: If you really like a job, but there is a detail that makes it not the right job for you, then don't give up until the employer knows what the issue may be. With a little brainstorming, many times this can be worked out.

15. "It's Not You . . . It's Me"

When to Walk

"I can guarantee you that money will not improve job satisfaction."

Realize that sometimes a job is not the job for you. At times we will attempt to fit a square peg in a round hole. We do this for many reasons. A large one is that the pay is good and we put ourselves in the position of the donkey chasing the carrot. I can guarantee you that money will not improve job satisfaction. Sometimes it is the location, it may be the time, or it may be the degree of stress or the wrong people. You do not want to sign on the bottom line for a job that you are unable to do. It is better to keep your professional respect than to go somewhere and not be able to fulfill your obligations. Remember there are other employers and employees.

 Mistake: Taking a job you know will not work out for both you and the employer.

Good Understanding

If you do walk away from a job where you have been negotiating to make it work and it doesn't, then make sure you walk away with a good understanding. On television and theater, you often see theatrics when a deal does not work. People give ultimatums, the suspense builds, the music gets louder, and then there is an outburst of anger and someone is devastated and has to face the repercussions of a damaged life by the decision. Well, as a physician, chances are that your negotiation will not work like this. It should not be that dramatic. It makes good for the movies, but you never want to terminate a negotiation during high emotion and anger. Many times a great chance at work does not work out for both parties. It is good to discuss why it didn't work out, but also this should be done in an amicable way.

You never know; an idea that works may come about hours, days, months, or years down the road. If they clearly understood your needs, they will keep you in mind just in case something else fits better. You also never know whom that job, hospital, or potential employer will mention your name to. I've even seen where one of the people attempting to negotiate may move to another company. They will keep you in mind as a good physician and may be able to do an agreement that will work for you in a different situation. The point is to make sure that you do not burn any bridges or blame the other party for why the negotiation did not work out. Just because it did not work out does not mean the other person or persons is now your enemy, nor does it mean it was not a good opportunity. Make sure it is clear to the employer why it will not work for you at this time.

 Conclusion: Be clear to yourself and the employer why the job will not work for you. People prefer honesty, and it keeps away questions. It is better to not start than to have to leave on bad terms.

16. "On Second Thought . . . It Is You"

"A noncompete agreement is an attempt by the employer to prevent an employee from competing for services and using trade secrets gained from employment."

 Mistake: Not realizing the best of intentions may go awry.

Non-compete Clauses

A non-compete agreement is an attempt by the employer to prevent an employee from competing for services and using trade secrets gained from employment. Non-compete clauses make sense in protecting the interest of a company from an employee.

Example

A large anesthesia practice has Dr. Johnson seeing patients at an outpatient surgical practice. Dr. Johnson is being paid a set salary by the anesthesia practice. Let's say the outpatient surgical facility is paying the anesthesia practice $250 per hour to have their facility covered, and Dr. Johnson is being paid by the anesthesia practice a yearly salary based at $185 per hour. Dr. Johnson then negotiates a deal where if they are willing to cut out the larger office, then he is willing to do the work for $200 per hour. So the issue is that the anesthesiologist did not find the work, but he used his insider knowledge in order to circumvent his employer.

Example

Another common issue is where several doctors work for a facility and decide to leave to start their own practice together. The newly formed group then actively recruits existing clients that were previously established with the other office. The group of physicians who left is taking all cash-paying patients with them as they start up their own office directly across the hall.

Non-compete clauses may be fashioned in several ways. Most often you see the dynamics of distance and time. Distance is typically judged in radius or diameter. Imagine if the radius is five miles of a particular clinic or hospital. The diameter of this is a total of ten miles. This measurement is not typically done by miles in routing on streets, but by the diameter straight lined from the building. Essentially, ten miles in diameter is wider than the great majority of American cities. This may cause a physician who is leaving to have to practice in another city. This becomes particularly an issue if the group has more than one office and the diameter includes the other offices. How long this stands is time limited. It often stands for one to two years. Another issue is that the non-compete clauses may stipulate that neither patients seen in the office nor previous office staff may go with the leaving physician to the next place of work. This may be extended to previous employer's group business contracts, affiliated hospitals, work agreements, and individual contractors.

Please note that all states have different laws regarding non-compete clauses where they are poorly supported to the exact opposite. Non-compete clauses tend to not have as much support if the clause keeps, or highly restricts, a physician from working. The issue is that breaking the non-compete clause can easily trigger a lawsuit and can be very costly. Remember that a large entity most likely has deeper pockets than an individual physician. Be careful before you sign and make sure you completely understand the non-compete clause and negotiate it out of the contract if you feel uncomfortable.

Termination

I live in Texas, which is a right-to-work state. Essentially, this means that individual employees do not have to pay dues or belong to unions. Unions are organizations that are formed to protect workers' rights and are often used to settle disputes between the employer and employees. Right to work is used here to mean that your job is not guaranteed and it does not protect the individual from unfair firing. It is important to pay particular attention to the termination clause in the contract because it lets you know how you may be terminated immediately. I've seen people get a job and not mention past issues that later cause immediate termination.

There are many common reasons for termination. Some of the immediate causes for termination are loss of a medical license, felony charges, loss of the ability to participate in Medicare/Medicaid, unsafe practice of medicine, mentally or physically unable to do the job, and lying on an application or leaving off information (such as criminal records or professional reprimands). Other issues include not showing up to work, fraudulent billing activity, belligerent behavior with staff, sexual misconduct, and substance abuse. Many employers will have provisions on how to handle these issues, and there may be protection under the code of conduct, but if the behavior is egregious, then it may still result in termination.

It is best to avoid these things by being professional about how you do your work. At the same time, the unexpected may occur. Some of this is spelled out in the contract and others may not be. If you run into a problem on the job, make sure you know what your rights are if the employer has a code of conduct. Now, it would be odd to an employer if, while interviewing or during recruitment of a physician, the physician asks, "What is the consequence of arriving to your shift late?" Another would be, "What is allowed under your substance abuse policy?" Of course, these things would cause an immediate red flag to your employer.

 Conclusion: Make sure there is a clean break in that unfortunate and unintended things happen. It is important to realize that two people working together for the rest of their lives is something that is not likely to happen. You want to plan the separation at the beginning rather than the end.

V.

Special Populations and Resources

17. Special Populations

Women

You can clearly see in medicine that numerically the number of male to female physicians is moving closer to one to one, and it is further estimated that soon there will be more female physicians than males. Even though more women are going to college and are increasingly the primary breadwinner in their homes, many find that they are still the person who is primarily in charge of childrearing and serve as the chief operational engineer of the home. This situation can cause a dichotomy with the professional desire to advance in your career as a physician and at the same time raise children and be a domestic engineer. This is even further exacerbated if the physician is single with children or has a husband who does not actively participate. Increasingly, you are also seeing men in single parent roles as well. At times, it may seem as if neither the career nor the home is to the best of expectations, thus leading to being overly critical. This can cause a back-and-forth juxtaposition with neither side seemingly winning or receiving self-satisfaction. With these factors occurring, the contract negotiations and job search are greatly affected.

 Mistake: Not considering that everyone's situation is unique and may have unanticipated demands and stressors.

A few factors to consider are after-school care, work hours, work demands, call coverage, and consistency of hours. These factors can limit the number and types of positions that are available. A high-paying job that requires sixty to seventy hours per week, with an unpredictable in-house call schedule, may not be ideal unless you have a stable support system as backup to a hectic and unpredictable day.

At the same time, a job with flexibility may be a good fit, such as a doctor working an inpatient unit with an eight-hour day. (Realize that with inpatient care, the patients are in the facility and are not as much on a time schedule than an outpatient clinic. So, essentially, rounding is done at the opportune time the physician sets as long as all the patients are seen and their needs are met.) Another option is a job that is consistent with time. The job may be that it is an eight-to-five repetitive schedule, and this even can work out well with a call schedule if the schedule is consistent. It is also good to know if the particular placement has a child care facility. You may find this at many of your larger hospital or university settings. If so, is there a waiting list? How long is the waiting list? What is the cost of child care in the area? This varies from city to city and within the same city. Realize, though, that given the two above examples, there are many female physicians who are working long and tenuous hours while maintaining healthy families and relationships.

Networking and Non-traditional Settings

If two people of the same sex are negotiating, negotiations may occur in a non-traditional and relaxed setting. These settings can be on a golf course, at a ball game, or in a local bar or eatery. These types of settings give an advantage to friends of people hiring and inside knowledge of positions that are open or may open soon.

Example

A male doctor is interviewing for a position with the male local hospital CEO at the end of the day. The two had a previous friendship outside of work as golfing buddies and both are fans of the local college basketball team where they both went to college. The CEO schedules an interview weeks in advance, without knowing their team would make it to the basketball tournament. As they are going through their discussion, they converse over how the game is going. The CEO then suggests they finish up at the bar down the street and catch the end of the game. It would be probable that the male CEO interviewer is less inclined to ask a woman the same due to fear of poor intentions. This type of request could be easily misconstrued when asking someone of the opposite sex to dinner when they are looking for employment. The contrast to this is going for a bite to eat and drinks gives both the CEO and the interviewee an opportunity to further discuss working out a win-win negotiation.

Single and Dating

Often we are seeing increasing numbers of unmarried young professional physicians. If a person is single and actively looking for a spouse, the person may seek employment in an urban area where there are more potential dating opportunities.

Disparities in Pay

"People may fear the perception of a woman going through a hard negotiation may cause her to be looked at differently from her male colleagues who do the same."

It has been shown in multiple studies that women make less than their male counterparts. Often this is assumed to occur due to women being more likely to work part time and being less likely to desire positions of leadership. The issue is that even when adjusting for hours of work, volume, and payer status of patients, female physicians make as much as 20 percent less than their male peers. Often when promotions occur within the department and other opportunities for an increased salary occur (like medical directorships), males are placed into these positions, which often have financial stipends attached.

Some of this can be explained through sexism in the workplace, where people feel men are more valuable as physicians or that you can lowball on the offer to women and they will accept the pay. There is even suggestion that women expect to be underpaid. Remember that people making decisions of physician pay are not always male, and often these sexist assumptions of pay are shared by both sexes and not just males. Other reasons are that many women are not as likely to feel comfortable with confrontation. In order to avoid confrontation, many women will defer negotiating and receive less salary. People may fear that the perception of a woman going through a hard negotiation may cause her to be looked at differently from her male colleagues who do the same. I would say that most people hiring should be well beyond this, but of course you can't predict everyone's thoughts.

Regardless of perception, remember that the contract has to be negotiated, and you don't want to sign something just to avoid difficult discussions. If you feel you are being undervalued and lowballed on an offer, I would recommend using hard numbers and research to show why a person of your qualifications, years of experience, work habits, and expertise deserves X amount of salary. Arguing the point without figures can appear highly opinionated with neither side seeing the other side's point.

Example

Dr. Kimberly Smith is interviewing at City Hospital. At the interview, she is offered a written contract with a salary of $185,000 per year. After doing her research on the average salary for her specialty, she sees that the average pay of a physician with her credentials, board certifications, and fifteen years of experience is $205,000 per year. In addition to this, she sees that in a medical professional newsletter, the hospital has a listed salary offer of $210,000. Dr. Smith has decided that she really likes the job and wants to take it, but she is unwilling to take 10 to 15 percent less than the going salary in the area. Dr. Smith went back to City

Hospital and noted that she saw the offer was much less than the listed price and less than the average salary in the area. She asked whether this was the correct or best offer or whether this was an oversight of City Hospital.

This should be enough in itself to get the salary higher. If City Hospital refuses to increase the offer, then it warrants a written letter requesting an explanation of why the physician received a contract offer with a lower salary than listed. It is important to not undervalue yourself because if you do, expect that others will view you the same.

Minorities

Minority physicians are a growing population of physicians in the United States. However, despite the increasing number of minorities in the United States, blacks and Hispanics have less representation as physicians than in the population. Black males inconsistently make less than white male counterparts, depending on setting and specialty. However, females consistently make less, and the disparity grows higher for black female physicians in comparison to their white male counterparts even when adjusted for workload, patient volume, and credentials, according to "How do Race and Sex Affect the Earnings of Primary Care Physicians" by William Weeks, et al. Hispanic and Asian physicians also show a disparity in salaries to their white counterparts. But unlike the differences in pay with blacks that have held consistent, their disparities in pay are diminishing. Also, there continues to be disparities in the number of people of color holding positions and receiving research, private, and public funds. Leadership positions, and in leadership within training institutions and universities, show disparities, as well.

Of course, you have some employers who make the conscious decision to not offer positions or the same income to people of color. I would more likely say this is done unconsciously in that the minority physician is offered less money due to the unconscious thoughts of the potential employer. The unconscious thought is that the value is not the same. It could also be that non-whites are less likely to negotiate for more and expect to be paid less. It is common that people who hire others may already know the person or know of the person due to their social circles. With most people who own large businesses being white, you find that their social constructs tend to be with more whites. This often leaves people of color on the outside looking in when it comes to highly sought-after jobs and positions. It is important that ethnic minorities engage in professional organizations and networking opportunities. Often contracts are negotiated, decisions are made, and people are hired in their own personal circles well before a formal interview or job listing has occurred.

 Conclusion: Everyone has unique circumstances that may impact employment. A good opportunity may not be great for your particular situation. The culture of diversity and tolerance, or lack thereof, in the workplace can make or break a job situation.

18. Academia

Many of us will choose a career in academics. When considering a contract in academia, you have to understand that there is a definite hierarchy process involved in moving your career forward. This is most often stated in the faculty handbook. Not only do you want to understand the written rules of advancement, but also the unwritten culture of where you are working. It is not only central to talk to the leadership of the department, but also junior faculty and those who are a few steps ahead of you in their academic careers. They will be more in tune to the culture of the department and are full of insight on the process of career advancement and will let you know if they feel the process is fair.

 Mistake: Thinking that working hard in an academic setting will make you a full professor quickly.

Generally, in all academic settings, you will have to start from the lower level of hierarchy, unless you have already advanced your career elsewhere and mostly in academia. Entry-level positions include instructor, lecturer, adjunct professor, and/or clinical associate. These types of positions may have a salary or they may be voluntary. Although the names can vary, often the starting junior faculty position is stated as assistant professor. The next level is associate professor, with the top position being full or tenured professor. Typically,

moving up the ladder will have to do with time and most importantly production. This is why it is important to know what the focus of
the particular institution is. Essentially, every department chair and
division chief likes the person who produces money and supports
their own salary. As the saying goes, "If it doesn't make money, it
doesn't make sense." It is difficult to see the benefit of someone who
is costing the department money and not contributing in return.

Many institutions will have opportunities for fast tracking, but those
goals need to be clearly defined. You want to make sure they are at-
tainable. When setting lofty goals, it is important to make sure that
you have the ability to attain them with institutional support and
individual ability to get the job done.

Pay attention to the needs of the institution and its emphasis. If gene
therapy research is your interest, but the academic center is heavy in
community outreach and receives large government grants to deliver
such services, then you may not be able to locate the resources needed to advance your focus of study. If you do decide to work there,
then there needs to be some understanding of how you will be supported in your interest. If not, you may either be set up for failure or
soon find that you need to change your career interest.

Realize that the more productive you are, the more likely you are
to move up the academic ladder. The opposite is true, as well. You
want to make yourself valuable to the institution and find your niche
within your community of professionals. Essentially, your *track* is
your primary financial support of the work you do. The most common tracks are academic and teaching, research, clinical duties, and
contracts. If you are on a research track, then your primary support
and income will be from research. If you are on an academic track,
then your primary support will be from funds for teaching, so forth
and so on.

If your research grant is supporting 50 percent of your salary and
the local county clinic is supporting the other 50 percent, and your
grant is for two years, then in two years you will lose half of your
financial support. In this case, you have to take a close look at where

you are going to be in two years on your research and how are you going to find another financial support for the other 50 percent of your salary. Clinicians may teach and do research, but if the primary focus of your track is clinical work, then your primary financial support is through billing for clinical work. If you are on that track, it is important to make sure that the institution where you are working is able to collect on billing. You can see a high volume of patients, but if they are unable to collect, then your hard work may quickly be overlooked, even though your inability to support your salary may be well beyond your control.

 Conclusion: If it is your goal to make full or tenured professor, understand that you must have a plan from the outset and a clear path to get to your goal.

19. Resources

Physician Recruiting Firms

There are many physician recruiting firms. Typically, they connect the job seeker to the job hiring company. They serve as the middle man. They normally have a job listing bank and attempt to combine the physician to a potential job that fulfills the physician and employer's needs. They can be very helpful in doing this.

Remember that the recruiting firm is working for you . . . and the potential employer. Understand that the firm is there to help both parties come to an agreement. Also understand that the recruiter and the recruiting firm receive a healthy compensation for getting you to sign on the bottom line. This also means that when it comes to the contract, the recruiter's interest is theirs first and both parties are second. They want to get the deal done. In saying this, remember that you are not their primary interest and that their recruiter could be "working the other side of the coin" or working as a double agent per se. This becomes an issue when the recruiter doesn't make money until you sign the contract. It can be helpful in that the recruitment company may ask the employer to make concessions for you to sign, but also they may ask the same of you. This is much like a mediator in that they are negotiating to get two parties in agreement. Unlike a mediator, who should be impartial to any particular side, a recruiting firm is partial to themselves. Also, a recruiter may be partial because they are hired by the potential employer to find them the best doctor at the best rate.

 Mistake: Not realizing that you may not be the recruiter's primary interest.

 Mistake: Thinking that because someone is a lawyer, they understand medical contract negotiations.

Medical Lawyers

> "The medical contract lawyer needs to be able to pick up on the issues of time and intensity of the service."

Medical lawyers are very beneficial in helping negotiate a contract because many contracts can have legal jargon that is difficult to understand. They are trained to pay attention to the details of the contract and catch things we may otherwise miss. You really want to make sure that the lawyer doing this has experience in medical contracts.

The reason I say this is that many times a non-physician may not clearly understand the type of job in the manner of intensity as length of work described in the contract. A job may say eight a.m. to five p.m. Imagine an outpatient job that says that it has an eight a.m. to five p.m. schedule and a maximum of forty scheduled patients per day, but you also you learn that the clinic advertises itself as a walk-in clinic, acute care facility with a policy of "no patient is turned away." The medical contract lawyer needs to be able to pick up on the issues of time and intensity of the service. You definitely need to know what the average number of walk-ins per day is. If that is two per day, then it may not be an issue, but if they are averaging twenty or more and do not limit how many and how late in the day they may come in, it can be safe to assume that you will be there after five p.m. This can make your day highly unpredictable and drive up job stress. The other question is how acute "acute care" is. What is the policy of sending patients to a more intensive setting? Many jobs look the same on paper, but the experiences may be very different depending upon volume and intensity, which may not be clearly defined in the contract.

 Conclusion: It is up to you to determine the best job for you. Other people will have their own ideas with their own interest at heart. Make sure their interest meets yours and not the other way around.

20. Private Practice And Entrepreneurship

Starting a Private Practice

"Business is simple—'Make more money than you spend.'"

The biggest question you want to ask before starting a private practice is: Do you want to own a business? Private practice is entrepreneurship. If you don't want to be a business owner, then you don't want to start a private practice. Just like some people have a barbershop, nail shop, car shop, beauty shop, bicycle shop, or tire shop, I have a psych shop. So, even though my professional title is a "psychiatrist," running the business is a major part of what is required. In medicine we are trained twelve to seventeen years post-high school on the practice of medicine. With our extensive training, we can essentially do it in our sleep. It is odd that for a majority of physicians, we are not trained on running a business in the profession that we are so highly skilled. Even though the majority of my day is spent seeing patients, the issue of running a business is just as mentally time consuming and draining.

 Mistake: Not realizing that owning a private practice is a business.

It is essential to have a good office manager and someone you can trust. My mother was my office manager. Well, too often I hear of mismanagement and theft of hundreds of thousands of dollars from doctors' offices. This occurs quite easily because as the owner/doctor, you are very busy with generating income for the office and it causes you to have to trust those working with you. At the same time, you have to keep a watchful eye on your money.

Also, having a good accountant is a must. You have to pay your taxes. Many do not know how many taxes are required of a business owner. I have found that it is important to make sure you understand as much about taxes as possible. The more you know, the more your accountant will be able to help you and keep you out of trouble. Payroll, school, individual, business, city, county, and state taxes add up quickly with interest and penalties if you unfortunately ever get behind.

Employee issues of hiring, firing, upsizing, and downsizing can be especially time consuming. Handling patient (customer) complaints regarding business operations and employee issues are things we are not trained for. As a business (practice) owner, you may find yourself being the CEO, president, secretary, treasurer, chief financial officer, operations manager, financial analyst, financial forecaster, director of business development, trainer, or whatever else may be required at the time.

It is important to understand that these roles can be very time consuming. Starting off, it is very time consuming and you need to be prepared to put the time in. Getting your paper work, forms, computers, and billing apparatus up, whether it is done in-house or outsourced, needs to be planned out with the expectation that it is completed whenever the job is done. There is no time limit or constraints when birthing a business or keeping it afloat. The time is "whatever it takes."

There are other ways to start in private practice, as well. Many people will start by being subsidized by a hospital or a large group. Essentially, another entity will give a salary for one to three years in exchange for your services. These companies make money by requiring the physician use their services. These services may include taking on and admitting inpatients at their hospital and using their lab, imaging, and ancillary services. Understand that these other services the doctor is doing most times pay more than your salary because the doctor essentially makes money by seeing patients, but the other services or other sources of income offset the cost of the physician.

An example of subsidizing your salary is to say that your salary is based on $15,000 per month and your year under this contract starts in January. The first month that you start, you only generated $5,000, then the entity subsidizing pays you the other $10,000. Assume by July of that same year you generate $12,000 per month, and then the hospital will pay you $3,000 to subsidize. Then by September you generate $15,000 plus until the end of the year. At this time the hospital does not have to subsidize you any further. The question then becomes who the money belongs to once you generate well over the subsidized amount.

Another option is to join a private group that is already up and functioning. This way you are able to avoid the birthing process of a practice because it is already set up and ready to go. These types of practices may pay a salary, you may pay a monthly fee for services, equally or unequally share the administrative cost, sublet space, or it may pay you a percentage of the income you generate for the practice minus the cost of running the practice. There are many details to consider with all of the above options. It is best to make sure you discuss these options during the contract negotiating and well before signing.

Another wrinkle to the fold is that many contracts can be verbal with no one ever signing anything. I would not recommend doing this, but I've seen it done with disastrous and sometimes great results. I would not take the chance.

How I Started My Practice

I started my practice by a combination of things. First, I had saved money in a retirement account when I was in residency and I did have a short stint teaching between undergrad and starting residency. I cashed out what I had saved with both. Most financial advisors would not recommend doing so, especially if your "financial advisor" sold you the mutual fund or annuity. (Understand that cashing out does incur cost and taxes that must be paid.) I figured that it was worth it to cash out $20,000 to make $150,000 in my first year out. I also borrowed money from my mother. (Thanks, Ma!) She did get her money back with interest . . . well, at least most of it. She also became my office manager. We used to debate over how this occurred, but if you finance the operation, you get to pick what you want to do. According to her, I begged her to come out of retirement as a counselor and take the job. Well, Mom's story always wins! I also had help from most of family along the way. (Thanks, fam!) We are truly a family-run business. I also have hired people who are not biological family, but I consider them family, as well.

During building the business and patients, I used other means to generate income. One way I did this was by working at a local hospital (taking a maximum of four inpatients per day), working at a residential hospital, doing consults at a local medical/surgical facility, and doing outpatient clinic work at two different facilities. When I started, I was working in my office approximately one and a half days per week. Many of these jobs would be considered contract work or moonlighting. As my office grew and required more time, I cut back on the other services and spent more time in my office. This eventually eased the transition I had into private practice and gave me time to grow it slowly and not be pressured into making the office my primary source of income on day one.

When I first started, I was not sure of how or what to do. I looked for office space. I based my space on where I expected to live in the city and where was there a need for physicians. I found a location and compared prices. I did not end up in the city I intended to be in. The rent prices and available space did not fit in my business plan. Next I needed a phone and Internet services. I had a referral from a family member to run lines and cables in my office space. I looked around for office furniture. I wanted to make sure the furniture fit the clients that I would be seeing and wanted to make sure the patients had a comfortable environment. Honestly, on day one I did not know how to find patients or how to bill for the patients I saw. My first patient came from a program that I was working with that needed outpatient services. The next one was referred by a family member. When I first started, I saw one patient a week for the first two weeks, then it was one patient a day by the third week, one patient an hour by the first month, and by week six and within the first three months, we were full with seeing twenty patient hours per week. We grew from me as an individual private practice to one of the largest practices in the fourth largest city in the US in the matter of five years.

 Conclusion: Starting a private practice is business entrepreneurship. Whether your practice is financially secure has little to do with your knowledge of medicine. It has more to do with your business acumen.

21. Reading Is Fundamental

Read the Contract!

Even though this seems very simple, it is odd how often people never read the contract they sign. The most important person who needs the contract is you . . . the person signing it. It is a lot more difficult to get out of a contract once you have signed it, showing that you are in legal agreement with the terms. By reading the contract yourself, you can help others who are reading it to understand what the contract is lacking. It also helps if you have someone you trust read the contract, as well, and give their opinion. I consult my colleagues regarding job and career questions all the time. One of the last things an employer wants from an employee is someone who agreed to do a contract and obviously can't fulfill the terms. Additionally, you do not want to be obligated to a job that you refuse or are unable to do.

 Mistake: Not reading the final contract before signing.

Necessary Changes

Make sure you contact the employer if there are things you are uncomfortable with in the contract. Many things are left to interpretation, so if you are unsure, get clarity. It is good to go over this verbally, but make sure the contract shows clarity of the issue. Simply drawing a line through and rewriting what you want is sufficient only to identify the areas that you are uncomfortable with. Realize that writing in what you want and initialing can mean absolutely nothing unless the other party did the same. Even at that, it is best to not sign until the document is retyped with the changes. Be sure to reread for the changes. I've seen well too many times where changes were discussed and verbally agreed upon and the contract came back unchanged.

 Conclusion: Read the final contract and make sure all negotiated changes are made.